SHE'S ALRIGHT

One Woman's Journey Through

Breast Cancer During Pregnancy

Robin Kimple Ellis

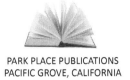

PARK PLACE PUBLICATIONS
PACIFIC GROVE, CALIFORNIA

She's Alright
Robin Kimple Ellis

© 2012 Robin Kimple Ellis

First Edition February 2012

ISBN 13: 978-1-935530-57-2

Front and back cover photos by Anne Staveley

Published by
Park Place Publications
Pacific Grove, California
www.parkplacepublications.com

Printed in Mexico

To order copies of this book:
www.shes-alright.com

Acknowledgements

For our daughter, Tess Elizabeth,
who is, by all accounts, a living miracle.
And for my husband Rich and our daughter Avery Nicole,
because when one of us has cancer, we all do.

And for Jenny Bird for giving me the title to this book,
for her steadfast and loyal friendship, for her propensity
with words and for always, always knowing just what to do,
just what to say and exactly how to say it.

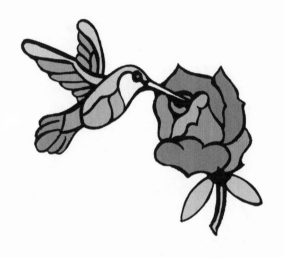

CONTENTS

CHAPTER 1

The Door

We pulled up in the parking lot of the medical building and managed to bring our large SUV to rest in a space designed for a compact. I put my hand on the door handle, paused, took a deep breath and rested my hand on my lap again. My husband noticed my reluctance to open the car door and stretched his hand over to my bare, freckled shoulder to comfort me. I stared down at the dashboard, mulling it over and over again in my mind. This was the day of days, the one I had been dreading since the diagnosis. I wanted Rich to pull the car out of the parking lot and drive. Just drive. Drive away from the fear and the unknowing. Drive away from the pathetic look on our friends' faces that we so often saw when they were trying their hardest to act "naturally." Drive away from the needles and the poison, from the CAT Scans and the X-Rays, from the blood tests and the fear.

"We've talked about this for so long now, Honey, and here it is. This is it! Don't be scared. I'll be right beside you all the way," he said to me. "Don't worry, Babe. We can do this."

"I'm not so sure I can. I thought I could, but now I'm not so sure," I said, my voice shaking. I raised my hand to my forehead and, with my thumb on my right eyebrow, stroked my newly-formed worry lines with my remaining fingers. Back and forth. Back and forth. I ran my fingers through my short, red curls. Then I took both of my hands and buried them deep in my hair, mussing it all up, my hair shaking and bouncing back into place, doing everything that good curly hair is destined to do. Then the tears burned my eyes. I blinked them back and pitched my head backward so that the tears would go back into my eyes. I took another deep breath, playing now with the ends of my short, bobbed hair, and thought about Jona.

Jona was a dear friend. We recognized each other as soul sisters the very first time we met. We even looked a little bit alike, if you could overlook the fact that Jona weighed 110 pounds soaking wet and I, on a good day, would have to lie down flat on my bed to squeeze my ample thighs and bum into my size 10 jeans! Otherwise we were very similar. Our hair was almost identical in its long, flowing curls that reached the middle of our backs. We were stunning, or so they used to tell us, our hair our very best feature. We both had bright blue eyes and joyful smiles. We were both cool and street smart, wise and wild, well dressed and well suited to our Southwestern environment. We partied hard, loved deeply and were loyal to the death. We made pasta and drank wine late into the night, smoking American Spirit cigarettes and talking expressively and excitedly knee to knee. We listened to Joni Mitchell and cried for her lost loves. We were there for each other at the birth of our children and sobbed joyfully, one for the other, as we witnessed the first look shared between mother and her baby—that bittersweet, magical moment of separation—one soul moving into two. We were true friends, and we loved each other.

A few weeks earlier, Jona had showed up unannounced at our house in Santa Fe. Her arrival had prodded me out of my robot-like state, albeit temporarily. Since the beginning of my cancer journey I had gone deep within myself. I would perform my daily tasks: the shopping, the cooking, tending to my husband and our toddler daughter. Everything looked pretty normal from the outside looking in. But if you knew me you could easily see how different I was. I was lost in a sea of fear and indecision and was rarely able to be anything but that: lost.

When I heard a car pull into the gravel driveway I thought it was Rich and our daughter Avery returning home, but I soon heard Jona's voice announcing her arrival, and I jumped up to greet her. And there she was, standing in the driveway wearing a hideous platinum blonde wig, with the silvery-yellow hair hanging all the way down to her behind. I was flabbergasted! Her saunter into the house was fun, light and full of humor, and I realized instantly that my good pal was just pulling a prank on me. "A bit of humor to lighten up the vibe, no doubt," I thought. Jona was always able to assign a happy face and a bit of hope to an otherwise heavy and hopeless situation. NOTHING could get that girl down.

I went up to my dear friend in her frightening "Frederick's of Hollywood" platinum wig to give her a big hug. I was truly happy to see her and happy to be rid of the darkness that surrounded me, even if it was just for a moment. As I approached her, Jona gently put her hand up on top of her head, motioned for me to pause for a moment, and then she did it. Jona pulled that tacky old wig off of her head, and in a rush of disbelief and confusion I realized what I was looking at on top of my good friend's head. Nothing. I was looking at absolutely nothing. Jona had shaved her head. She had shaved all of her beautiful hair off of her head. Her beautifully shaped scalp shined like polished marble. I was dumbfounded. I dropped to my knees in the midst of a whirlwind of shock and confusion, grasping at the slim thread of a vague understanding of what I was seeing, hoping that that slim thread might be sturdy enough for me to pull myself up on—pull myself back into my mind and body and some semblance of sanity. At that very moment, Jona joined me down on the kitchen floor, grabbed my hands and, with tears in her eyes and a steady voice said, "Robin..... How can I say, 'Oh honey, it's just hair. It's no big deal. Don't be sad.......' if I still have mine?"

Jona and I sat on the kitchen floor in my haunted house in Santa Fe and wept and cried and sobbed with each other. I was filled with a mixture of shock and awe and disbelief. But there was something else I felt, too. Something strange and foreign to me. So foreign in fact that I didn't know WHAT the feeling was. Then I realized what this strange sensation was. This strange sensation that I was experiencing in my body, mind and spirit all at the same time was, simply, selflessness. Pure selflessness. I was in the presence of a human being who was, at that very moment, creating a Holy Space. A sacred moment of pure, unconditional love shared between two beings. The space shared by the two of us, there on the kitchen floor was a HOLY PLACE: as holy as Lourdes or the hill on Calvary, as sacred as the Dome of the Rock and the Garden of Gethsemane. As sacred as the sound of your baby's first cry.

⊡ ⊡ ⊡

"Robin, honey, it's time to go in. We're a little bit late as it is," Rich said as he placed his hand calmly and lovingly on my shoulder. My husband's words drew me back into my body, back from the memory of the kitchen floor and the holy moment I had shared with my friend. Now I was squarely back in the passenger seat of our SUV, face red from sobbing, eyes puffy and sunken in from too many sleepless nights and fearful days. It was time to go. I took a deep breath and reached for the door handle, opened it and stepped down to the asphalt. Rich followed suit and we walked toward the entrance of the cancer center hand in hand.

Our footsteps were slow and heavy, as if our bodies weighed a thousand pounds a piece. Finally the clear, swinging doors were in front of us. "NEW MEXICO CANCER CARE" written on the glass with the names of a dozen doctors and their business hours. Normal things to read on a normal door of some normal business or doctor's office, but this door was no ordinary door. This door was THE door. And there it was, right in front of us. I reached out for the door handle, but I couldn't open it. I stood there in front of the door, my hand quivering, trying with everything in me to reach out and pull that door open. But I just couldn't. I had to step back into the shadows underneath a stairwell and sob. I sobbed and sobbed and sobbed on my husband's shoulder, and he just held me as I cried. After what seemed like an eternity to me, the crying subsided a bit. I was still gasping for little in-breaths uncontrollably, like a young child who has just had a nice, long, tantrum-driven cry. I was inadvertently gasping for little breaths of air, unable to control the aftereffects of a total breakdown; I composed myself once again and walked to the door. This time my hand was able to grab the handle, pull it open and walk inside.

The nursing staff greeted us both and asked us to sit down and fill out the usual paperwork and as we were just finishing the last form on the clipboard, I heard my name called. The medical nurse was in the front lobby calling my name, ready to walk me back to the doctor's office and the chemo room. Try as I might, I COULD NOT hold back the tears as we walked the labyrinth of hallways back to Dr. Lopez' office. Once there, I was escorted in to a seat on a comfy leather chair as Rich trailed after me. If any real information was discussed during the 10 minutes in

Dr. Lopez' office I had no recollection of it. It looked and sounded like an hallucination, not real life. I heard nothing, understood nothing, said nothing at all. Suddenly the doctor and my husband stood up and I was turned over to the care of one of the chemo nurses. She escorted me into a room filled with leatherette lazy-boy chairs sitting in a circle. In these chairs were sitting some very sick people, all with wires and tubes sticking into their veins and lots of noisy machines surrounding them. Some of them attempted a smile. Most had their eyes closed, living in a quiet world of their own; coping as best they could.

The nurse ushered me over to my own chair where I was told to sit down and relax and to not be scared. I was able to obey the first of those three commands. The other two were lost to me; unreachable. The tears began to flow again, a little more controlled this time. I looked over to the man sitting in the chair in the corner. Most of his face had been surgically removed and it was shocking and difficult to keep his gaze. But he looked at me, with tubes full of poison running into him and half of his face removed, looking more like a monster than a man. He looked at me with bright, shining eyes, managed a mangled smile with his now-deformed mouth, and uttered softly, like he was sharing a precious secret with me, "Don't be scared, sweetie. God's got it! You're gonna be just fine. I have a way of knowing these things."

I didn't say a word, but battled with my own tears as the nurse who administered the chemo pulled her little chair over by mine with all of the paraphernalia necessary for infusing chemo into someone's arm. She barely looked at me as she approached, concentrating mainly on all the bags and tubes and syringes that she was juggling. As she was able to negotiate the small supplies table next to me and deposit her load on to it, her eyes met mine. Just after our eyes met and she had introduced herself to me, she glanced down at my stomach. As she looked at my body and processed what she was seeing, the nurse's eyes got huge, and she excused herself and went straight over to Dr. Lopez who was standing just outside of the chemo room looking over a patient's chart.

The nurse, clearly panicked and speaking loudly enough for everyone in the office to hear, said, "Dr. Lopez, do you KNOW that this woman is pregnant? We can't administer chemotherapy to a pregnant woman! Are you SURE this is the right patient and the right chart?"

"Yes, she is the right patient, and you have the correct chart," the doctor retorted. "Our Robin is six months pregnant. And we begin her chemotherapy today."

CHAPTER 2

Hair

I've always fancied myself a spiritual person. As a matter of fact, when I was a child, I remembered God. I remembered how it felt to be with Him. I felt like I WAS with Him. He felt like a friend. He was a friend that was always with me but who I couldn't necessarily see. I didn't need to see Him. I knew He was there. Once when I was about five years old I was on a trip through the Rocky Mountains with my parents, sisters and my grandparents, Ma Maw and Pa Paw. We were driving in a two car convoy through a mountain pass in New Mexico, both cars towing Nimrod pop-up campers behind them, on our way to the Tres Ritos Campgrounds that my family loved to visit. I was riding in the car with Ma Maw and Pa Paw, and, in the twistiest, turniest part of the mountain pass it started to rain. No, it started to pour! A dark cloud had popped up out of nowhere like it so often does in those mountains, and the rain fell out of the sky so hard that you couldn't see the road through the windshield. At that point I, at five years old, started to pray out loud. I prayed, "God, please let it stop raining so that Pa Paw can see to drive." Well, the rain didn't stop right away, but I wasn't confused or disappointed. I told my grandparents, "Well, that's ok. I don't think that God could hear us because of the bad reception!" I knew He had heard my prayer, and the rain did finally stop. And Pa Paw could see to drive.

That kind of surety has been with me all through my life. I have a personal relationship with God that can neither be explained nor daunted. My God is great and can not be denied or doubted. From these truths I have navigated through this life—faithful that God Is, that I will always be in His loving care as will every creature that has ever been or will ever be.

Well, that being said, I have a confession to make. The confession can be summed up in one word. That word is HAIR.

Now, one would think that a *truly spiritual* person like myself with the direct line to the Creator of the Universe would, in fact, have some highly evolved take on this whole cancer thing. One would think that a person like me would ascertain some mystical, meaningful purpose for this tragic event in my life. Surely someone of my *expansive personal knowledge* of God Himself would take a calamitous misfortune like Stage 2 breast cancer during pregnancy and turn it into some unique opportunity to grow and serve the planet. From all of this *immensity of spirit*, all of the stuff which made me who I was—with a well grounded knowing and understanding of the great mysteries of life—and all I could think about was my hair. Yep, my hair. I was going to lose my hair. No doubt about it. All of it. Everywhere. Yes, even *down there!*

I was born with naturally curly hair. Now of course when I was younger, when I was a little girl, I thought it was a curse. The fashion of the day was hair that was long and board-straight, and blonde if you could swing it! And there I was, with light brown curls falling down around my face and shoulders. I thought I would die. In junior high I would wash my hair at night and sleep with a hat on my head so that when I woke up my hair would be plastered down around my face and hung down to my shoulders like a weathered piece of hard felt. It looked terrible, but at least it wasn't curly! Then the 80's happened. Glory Hallelujah! Big hair was IN! My last two years of high school, I gave up the vain practice of straightening my curls and, for the first time in my curly life, I was able to let my hair live out its destiny. I grew it long and learned about "product" which helped it to be even bigger and curlier than seemed humanly possible. I had come in to my own. Or at least my hair had. There's a saying in the South that says, "The bigger the hair, the closer you are to God." Well, I had sure enough 'got religion'! I was closer to God than anyone in my whole school! And I was, as far as my hair was concerned, happy at last. I had gratefully and joyfully arrived in Hair Heaven.

As the years rolled by and I came into my own, my hair became my crowning glory. I let my soft, brown curls grow down to the middle of my back and tinted it with hints of mahogany and gold. There was not a day that went by without someone commenting about my beautiful hair. I played with it and hid behind it. I flaunted it and flirted with it. It was my best feature, to be sure, and people began to know me by my hair. I WAS my hair. It totally defined me. Or so I thought.

When the cancer diagnosis had some time to sink in to my brain, as I began to accept it as the indisputable fact that it was, I began to think about chemo. And as I thought about chemo, I thought about my hair. I was going to lose my hair! My beautiful hair. Nothing I could do about it. No way I could change it. It was going to happen. And it was going to happen to me.

Oh, the despair. I was paralyzed with grief over the thought of being bald. I would look like all the other cancer freaks I had ever seen in pictures or in public—bald and sickly, looking like they had one foot in the grave. How could it be? How could this be happening to ME? But it was happening. And it was happening to ME. One day soon I would be bald, and there was NOTHING I could do about it.

Well, I cried and I cried and I cried some more. I cried with my husband and I cried with my friends. I cried until I thought I could cry no more. Then I came up with a plan. Now, losing your hair to chemotherapy takes all of your power away from you. The whole cancer experience does. You feel as if you've lost any and all control over your life and, in a way, you have. If you decide to listen to your doctors and follow the path that they prescribe for you it's like launching a ship into strange waters with someone besides you at the helm. You become suddenly and absolutely impotent. It's a peculiar sensation. Here you are an adult human being, having lived your life the way you choose since you left the care of your parents. You live where you choose, eat what you like, cook or don't cook, exercise or not, have lovers or don't. Your life is your own. The choices you make are yours alone, be them good or bad, for your benefit or to your detriment. AT LEAST you are in control. When you are diagnosed with cancer, your life is not your own anymore.

This whole new reality of powerlessness bothered me, to say the least. I had been stripped of my position as master and commander of my own destiny. Many times I sat, unable to move, defeated and deflated and barely able to breathe. Up to that point I'd been a person defined by her freedom and individuality, wild and free and unburdened by the tethers of worldly concerns and restraints. Now here I was, imprisoned by my circumstances. I was stuck in the world and the laws that govern it, and there was nowhere to run. Or was there?

I had a plan. I had one little trick left that was hidden way up my sleeve and I was getting excited about it! Perhaps I hadn't lost control of my destiny after all! "Who says I have to lose my hair?" I asked myself. "Where is it written that I have to be at the mercy of the doctors and their schedules? WHO said that THEY hold all of the cards? They're not the boss of me!!!!!!!" I had a plan. I had one last moment at the helm, steering my own ship, in control of my own life, master of my own destiny. I felt the power again! I felt like a child again alone on my bike for the very first time, riding steady and straight and fast all on my own. I was free! I had a choice to make that was mine and mine alone. It was my hair and I would choose what to do with it. I would choose its destiny. And so I did it. Before the first chemo, before the inevitable happened TO me and my hair started falling out in big clumps in the shower, I did it. I did it. It didn't DO me. I did it.....

I shaved my own head.

CHAPTER 3

The Freak

If light could bend you could see around corners. I don't know why this scientific fact fascinated me so much in my youth, but for me it was a real mind-bender. It's funny the things you remember. Out of all the years of education that I received, that one concept stands out to me more than any other. I wonder if it's because it is, in fact, true?

My cancer diagnosis hit me broadside. Totally T-Boned me. Never saw it coming. No one does. Cancer is a sneaky little bastard. It creeps up on you and surprises you when you least expect it, and it changes your whole life and the life of your family forever. I just happen to be one of the lucky ones that lived to tell the tale.

Let's face it, though. Cancer patients look terrible. They're scary looking. When I was still a healthy, innocent by-stander I was terrified of sick people. All I knew was that they LOOKED so bad. I never thought about how they felt. They didn't register on the radar as real human beings. They were just sick people—not alive, not yet dead. Just kind of there. WAY over there if I could manage it.

Then I became a cancer patient myself. When I joined the ranks of the bald, sick and scary, I got a different view of things to say the least.

Now I really must mention something about myself. I am NOT a wig person. I wanted to be a wig person, thought that I could be if I tried. I bought a few of them before I lost my hair, (and they weren't cheap!) All that said, I just hated them. Every time I put a wig on my bald head I felt like I was dressing up for Halloween, and I always hated Halloween. Plus, they were so itchy! I looked ridiculous and I felt like an imposter. So, needless to say, I didn't wear a lot of wigs during my bald days. What I ended up wearing were bandanas on top of my head, like a kind of a make-shift hat, but much more comfortable. So, I had my head covered when I went out in public. Well, sort of.

Then there's the facial hair. I'm not talking about the unfortunate mustaches and five o'clock shadows that my Southern European or Latin girlfriends have had to deal with all their lives. I'm talking about standard issue facial hair. I'm talking about eyebrows and eyelashes. They don't make wigs for those. Well, actually they DO make "wigs," as such, for eyebrows and eyelashes. And they do have make-up specifically made to draw those greasy little lines on your face that are supposed to look like eyebrows. But they don't. They look like greasy little lines on your face where your eyebrows SHOULD be. When I was a young girl they called fake eyelashes "falsies." I'd probably poke my eyeballs out trying to get one of those on my lashline.

Perhaps the picture is getting clearer for you, O reader. I'm not much of a girlie-girl. Not even the basic, simple stuff. I'm more of a natural girl. You might find me with a bit of blush and lipstick just to make myself feel fully "dressed," add a little light eyeliner and mascara to that equation for VERY special occasions, and that's about it for this kid. So the thought of actually applying these cosmetic "prosthetics" to my skull and face was a joke. I would have spent my days feeling like an actress on a stage covered in grease paint and wearing a costume that was three sizes too big. It just didn't work for me. I was doomed to walk the planet masquerading as just exactly what I was: a cancer patient.

◻ ◻ ◻

Now the grocery store was my beat. For a while there when we lived in Taos, it was my entire social life. I spent a lot of time shopping for food and chewing the fat with the other customers and the check-out girls. I had my favorites, of course. And there were those, too, who I avoided like the plague! Being the mother of a toddler, a trip to the grocery store was a good excuse to get out of the house, show off your baby and socialize a bit, especially when it's cold outside and the park is off limits. I mean, who doesn't love a good market? I found a great store in Santa Fe close to my house. It had big, wide aisles, clean new carts and a fresh veggie section that had its own little eco system. Every now and then as I was squeezing avocados and checking a pint of strawberries for the moldy ones at the bottom, a little spray of rain would fall over the produce. It even had a little sound track of soft, rolling thunder sounding out of clever little speakers hidden somewhere in the display case. How cool is that!

I LOVE grocery stores. I mean, who doesn't, right? They have everything you need and they're so pretty, too! Especially the big, swanky one in Santa Fe that I had discovered. I had found my new home, my hot new hangout. My daughter and I would shop 'till we dropped, enjoying every minute of our social outing and thoroughly satisfying my ancient instinct to "gather." Now why on earth was I grocery shopping in Santa Fe when we lived in Taos, you might ask? After I was diagnosed with breast cancer, my husband and I decided to move. I was desperate for a little anonymity and Santa Fe just made sense for us. Bless their hearts, no one in our little community, friend or foe, knew how to deal with my disease. No one knew what to say. Well, there were those who so generously shared stories of their Aunt Elsie who had cured her own cancer by eating ooma gooma berries or some such thing. Oh dear! I didn't know what to say and neither did they. So we packed it up and moved to the "Big City."

Aaaaaaaaaahhhhhhhhhh, the thriving metropolis of Santa Fe. Now I wouldn't be plagued by the sad, pathetic looks on our friends' faces or the crazy, wild stories of miraculous healings and cures. I was safe now. Anonymous. Able to go through my experience all on my own and without interference from friends or acquaintances, no matter how heartfelt and sincere they may had been. I was free now. Free to be me. Free to be a Cancer Patient in public. Free to be "The Freak."

If light could bend you could see around corners. But light CAN'T bend, and you CAN'T see around corners. Because if you could, you wouldn't believe it anyway.

I first noticed it in the grocery store. Where else, right? Perhaps I should paint the picture for you. Here was me: bald, pregnant, obviously sick and pushing a beautiful little toddler around in the baby seat of the grocery cart. Wow. What an image. On one knew what to make of me. No one could figure me out. And worse than anything, no one would make eye-contact with me. No one would engage. People were scared of me and gave me a wide berth, not wanting to touch me, not wanting to have to talk to me. Not wanting to ask me questions. Not wanting to "get any on them." It was heart-wrenching. I had spent my whole life talking to people, especially strangers. Strangers were my specialty. I had a gift of making people feel good, making them laugh, making them feel good about themselves. I had a gift of making people smile. I loved my gift and have always considered it a God-given talent.

Well, I couldn't use that gift anymore, because no one would get near me. I could feel people's eyes on me and as soon as I would look their direction, try to make eye contact, they would look away. They'd look at the floor, or re-arrange their groceries. They would do anything they could to keep from having to engage with me. I made them very uncomfortable. I mean, the tension was palpable. I wanted to scream out, "GO AHEAD AND ASK ME! I KNOW YOU WANT TO KNOW! I have a story. Ask me what it is!" But I didn't scream out. And they didn't ask. I was "The Freak" now. I was no longer an attractive young woman with something kind and witty to say. I was "The Freak," nothing more.

If light COULD bend and we could see around corners, I wouldn't have recognized myself or what I had become. No one paid attention to me anymore. They didn't see me. They only saw my disease. It was a sad and lonely planet that I lived on. Totally alone. Unapproachable. An untouchable.

Ever since that time in my life, I go out of my way to talk to cancer patients when I run into them in public. I ask them about their treatment and how they're feeling. I tell them not to lose hope. I talk to people in wheelchairs, too. EVERY chance I get. One thing I took away from that experience, as I peered into my own past, is a feeling of pure shame. How disgusted I was at myself for avoiding the sick and infirm members of my community for my entire life. I was just like them—the folks in the grocery store. I was scared of sick people and would do anything I could to avoid engaging with them. Yep, I had been "one of them." I will never be "one of them" again. Never.

Even those who look like freaks have a story. There's a story that needs to be told. And we need to be there to listen.

CHAPTER 4

Julie the Midwife

Taos has a lot of hippies. We're talking hippies of all types, shapes and sizes. Hippies from the very old to the very young. Clean hippies and stinky hippies. Hippies that are pretending that they're NOT hippies anymore, but they really are. Then there are those, too who are playing the hippie lifestyle 'cause they think it's cool. I kind of like hippies. I guess I AM a kind of pseudo-hippie, in a real loose sort of a way. I like to grow my own vegetables, I don't wear make up or style my hair all fussy, and I LOVE to shop at natural food markets. I mean, who doesn't, right? They're just so pretty inside, and you always feel just a little healthier when you shop there, don't you?

We lived in Taos with all those hippies when we found out we were pregnant with our first child. We were over the moon, as all young family-planning couples are when the test comes back with a little + instead of a -. It was the happiest day of our life. I was so happy I could have peed in little cups ALL DAY and it wouldn't have bothered me. We were going to have a baby. And we were going to do it in our beloved Taos.

Now, people in Taos have their own way of doing things. They have a radio station like most communities do, but theirs is solar powered. They build houses like they do in all communities, but theirs are made out of aluminum cans and tires. Well, some of them, anyway. They're called "Earth Ships" if you want to check them out. If they're not building their houses out of cans and tires they're making them out of adobe—which is another way of saying they build their houses out of mud. Don't get me wrong, I LOVE the architectural style native to New Mexico. My husband and I built a house of our own out of mud, and it was a unique work of art, to be sure. I love the 'different-ness' of Taos, New Mexico. Hell, that's why we lived there after all.

They have their own way of having babies in Taos, too. There is a very strong pull toward natural childbirth in the land of 'different-ness'. One hundred years of medical advancement and scientific marvels, (like anesthesia, for example!) are thrown along the wayside for the betterment of women and their babies during childbirth. There are some undeniable advantages to having your baby the 'natural' way: no pesky hospital rooms or nurses, no mysterious machines that go "bing" all through the day and night for no apparent reason, no ugly hospital gowns that don't close up in the back. I mean that's just evil! Who designed those things, anyway? To wear a hospital gown when your mass is similar to that of a beached walrus is humiliating to say the least! That is the one area of the body that you MOST want covered when you're about to give birth! Who thinks these things up, anyway?

Then there is the distinct disadvantage of going the 'natural' childbirth route. No pain meds. No help whatsoever with the excruciating agony of labor. Nope, not even an aspirin. I was begging for a shot of tequila toward the end of it all, no joke! Anything to make the pain go away. But oh no, not when you're having your baby 'naturally'. You just have to bite on a stick and deal.

It's not all bad, though. There are some parts of having your baby at home with a midwife that are quite wonderful. You are in your own comfy house with all your stuff around you. You can light candles and burn incense and, if you're lucky like me and your best friend is a world class singer-songwriter, you can have soft soothing music played for you to calm your frightened soul and to softly serenade your baby into this world. You can have your sweet husband there with you cheering you on and holding you up --- making it all seem possible—helping it all to make sense. Your whole family can be there with you as you labor, which was an amazing perk.

Natural childbirth is all very Zen. Well, potentially Zen, anyway. Let's just say that there are very definite Zen possibilities when you have your baby at home. Very natural. Very normal. Just like your grandmother and great-grandmother did it all those years ago. Our maternal ancestors had been biting on sticks and giving birth to babies for millennia. Now who was I to break with such a grand tradition! Plus, everyone else in Taos was doing it in the late 20th Century. So why shouldn't I? It seemed good, healthy and a perfect choice for the pseudo-hippie that I had become. So, my husband and I climbed on-board the Natural Childbirth Bandwagon, and away we went....

We did a little research into the best midwives in our area, and one came highly recommended by everyone we spoke with: Julie the Midwife. Our first meeting with Julie, we knew we had found a match. We loved her, she loved us, she was highly qualified and, as important as anything else to Rich and me she was cool. I've never met a person more perfect for her chosen profession. I mean, if you looked up the word "midwife" in the dictionary there would be a picture of Julie. She was smart, compassionate and totally dedicated to her 'calling'.

We signed on immediately with Julie the Midwife and began all of the pre-natal exams and birthing classes, read all the books she recommended and, before we knew it, it was time. I was enormous! I couldn't believe how much a human body could change when it was with child. When I saw pregnant women as a kid I always thought their bellies were soft and squishy like a pillow. Wrong! My belly was tight and taut as a trampoline, no room left in there for anything—even my lungs, it turns out. Towards the end of my pregnancy I had to sleep sitting up so I could breathe sufficiently enough to keep me alive through the night! All I could think of was, "How on earth do people carry twins?" I could barely manage with one!

So, my water broke. I was standing in our kitchen making spaghetti sauce and SPLASH! There was my water all over the kitchen floor. It was time! Or at least I thought it was. It took our baby another 48 hours to come out and meet us. The child was in no hurry at all. My labor pains started slowly and gently with the help of our doula (or birthing assistant). She worked on some pressure points on the balls of my feel and, as if by magic, my labor began. Oh, happy day! I just couldn't wait to see our baby for the first time, this little being who had been living and dancing inside of me for the last nine months. I had prayed for a baby all my life and this, at long last, was the holy moment when I could hold my baby for the very first time. Well, holy moment it was! But to GET to that actual holy moment took a lot longer and was a lot more intense than I could ever have possibly imagined! They don't tell you about the REAL stuff that happens during labor in birthing class. If they did everyone would run screaming out of the room! Hell, the husbands would undoubtedly be the first ones out the door! When I say that natural childbirth is intense, that is putting it very mildly. It's like a Civil War battle going on inside your body—the North against the South. The North represents your brain, the South represents your nether regions. There's a wave of chemicals from the North which sends the pain rolling down in to the South. The waves of pain seem like they're never going to stop, like the battle will never be won. But the battle is won, finally, and the South wins this war! That baby comes rolling out of the birth canal amidst the screaming and the groaning and the pushing and then, ever so gently, slips into the midwife's hands. Julie the Midwife took that baby of ours and put it right on my tummy. And that little baby had the bluest eyes I'd ever seen. And that little baby went right for it's first little meal of it's first little life of yummy, warm mommy milk. And the war was over, the battle was won, the pain was immediately forgotten, and all was well with the world.

There was one little thing, though. One tiny little issue that my husband and I had overlooked. Rich and I had decided that we didn't want to know if our baby was a boy or a girl until it was born. We thought that was pretty cool to wait and be surprised the day the baby arrived. And I have to tell you, I was 100% certain that our baby was a boy. He was strong and big and active in my stomach. The vibe was SO boy! We were so certain, in fact, that we had only come up with boys' names and had finally agreed that our baby was going to be named Ethan Hamilton Ellis. Beautiful name, right? Well, not so much for a girl, though..... Holy smokes, it's a GIRL! Our baby is a girl! How did that happen? I was so certain and, as it turns out, I was SO WRONG! What are we going to do now? We haven't even THOUGHT of girls names, much less agreed on one!

They do things differently in Taos, though. In Taos you can take all the time you want to name your baby. Well, they give you a month, but I think that's pretty nice of them, anyway. So, we thought and we prayed and we wondered. We asked our little baby girl, whispered right in her little ear, we said, "Hey! Hey baby! What's your name, anyway? Can you help us out a little bit here? Got any ideas? We sure don't, and we're in a bit of a predicament. What do you think about it all, baby?" She looked back at us with the bluest eyes we'd ever seen and said nothing. Absolutely nothing. Oh well. No help there….. Then I remembered a name I had seen in a baby name book. I had just barely even scanned the girls' names ever so slightly, because I just KNEW I was having a boy, right? I remembered the name Avery and how much I had liked it. Rich agreed. He had always liked the name Nicole, and I agreed. And so it happened. We named that little baby girl of ours (who was supposed to be a boy!). We named her Avery Nicole Ellis. So now the battle was over, the South had won, and someone had cleaned up the battlefield. We had our beautiful little baby in our arms, and she had a beautiful name, and all was well with the world. (That is, until we tried to get her in her little car seat for the first time! Who knew such a simple thing could be so complicated!!! I mean, we're educated people, right? Help!)

◙ ◙ ◙

Well, we got the hang of the whole car seat thing. Turned out it wasn't as complicated as we had imagined. Now, getting her into a pair of tiny white tights for a Christmas party was, I think, the hardest thing I've ever done in my entire life! Have you ever tried to put a two month old sweet baby girl into a pair of tiny tights? It's hilarious. Someone should do a comedy routine about it some day. Oh Lordy, the things young parents have to learn how to do! We learn how to get creative on the spot—whatever the situation calls for.

Time passed slowly with our new baby. It is the most magical time when you bring your baby home, get to know her, learn how to read her thoughts and anticipate her needs. We were madly in love with her, amazed and grateful to God for our little miracle.

We continued our visits with Julie the Midwife. They call it post-natal care and she tended to both me and baby Avery, making sure that she was well and growing as she should be, and taking care of my battle wounds as well, making sure I was healing "down there," making certain that my milk had come in and that Avery and I had conquered the art of breast feeding to our satisfaction. I, like most women, had better luck with one breast than the other. My right breast was full and plentiful whereas my left never quite engorged nor produced much milk. Oh well. She's fine with the one breast, and if my nipple doesn't fall off from being suckled so voraciously everything should be just fine, I always said.

Avery had just turned ten months old when we went back to see Julie the Midwife for yet another check-up. By this time we had become good friends, so it was always a pleasure to be cared for by her. This particular check-up she wanted to run some test on my urine. Well, God knows I know how to pee in a cup by now! Gotten pretty good at it as a matter of fact. So I did. I peed in a cup for Julie the Midwife with my ten month old toddler sitting on the floor playing with some colorful baby toy with colored blocks that you move around on a wire. She always loved those…. After about ten minutes Julie the Midwife came out of the lab, and her face was white as a sheet. "Uh oh," were the first words out of my mouth. "What is it, Julie? Is everything ok? Did I pee the wrong color? Is something wrong with my, uh, stuff down there? What is it?" She asked me to go into the lab with her so we could speak privately, which freaked me out even more. We got into the room, she swiveled around to face me, and was silent once again. "What is it, Julie? Is there something wrong with me?" She looked back at me and, with a sly smile, she said, "You're pregnant again, honey. Congratulations!" Oh-my-God. I'm pregnant again??? I felt like I was going to pass out. Literally. I mean, I wanted to have another child SOME day, but Oh My Gosh. Not now! I have a toddler who's barely walking and takes all of my time and attention and love and caring, and I have ANOTHER ONE COMING? Julie the Midwife sat me down and gave me a glass of water to drink. I took some deep breaths, in and out, in and out. I'm feeling calmer now. Another baby. Oh how lovely! How very wonderful! I'm going to have another baby. Breathe in. Breathe out. Find the Zen. Ahhhhhhh. There it is. I'm going to have another baby. I jumped up and gave Julie the Midwife a huge hug, and we giggled and laughed, arm in arm, all the way out to where baby Avery was playing with the colorful blocks on the wire that she loved so much. I picked her up off the floor and floated out of the birth center, my feet never touching the ground. "You're going to have a baby brother or sister, Avery! What do you think about that?" She wooed and cooed like babies do, I placed her in her little car seat (which was MUCH easier after ten months of practice!) and I started the car engine. I sat there for a moment and the thought hit me. Oh my gosh, what am I going to tell Rich?????????

Well, I'm here to tell you that smelling salts never should have been taken off the market! I could have used some the night I told Rich that we were pregnant again. But, like with me, the shock wore off quickly and was replaced by pure excitement. We're going to have another baby! I wonder what it'll look like? Will it be like her sister, blonde haired and blue eyed and brilliant? Maybe it'll be a boy this time. And we talked and talked and asked a million rhetorical, unanswerable questions until it was well into the night and our baby Avery had fallen asleep between us, ignoring our high, excitable tones and animated gestures. Not long after Avery fell asleep, Rich and I did, too. We were exhausted from the fear and excitement and joy. We, the three of us, slept deeply and soundly together until the birds began chirping and the sun shined in the new morning.

◻ ◻ ◻

We were back in Julie the Midwife's care for baby number two. And yes, Rich and I decided on natural childbirth again. (How soon we forget, right?) We made it past the first few pre-natal exams and flew through the first trimester with no problems at all. Well, there was that pesky old morning sickness thing which I got in the evenings, instead. (Always the rebel!) But besides that most common of all symptoms of early pregnancy, everything was good and all was well with the world.

Before we knew it we were half way through our 2nd trimester—right at 4 ½ months, and we were off for our pre-natal check-up. Julie the Midwife did all the normal things, listened to my heartbeat, then to the baby's heartbeat, took my pulse and my blood pressure. Gave me a breast exam. All the usual things. When she was examining my left breast, she spent an inordinate amount of time feeling around one part of it. Kept rubbing it and putting pressure on it, making little circles with her fingers like she always did. I looked up at her face and there were worry lines between her eyebrows. She looked concerned. "What's up Julie? Do I have a clogged milk duct or something? There's all kinds of activity in my breasts right now. They're changing all the time!" "Well, it might be a clogged milk duct, but I don't think so. I don't like the way this lump feels." As she's talking she continued to investigate it with her fingertips, and the worried look never left her face. "We'll take a look at that again next month at your pre-natal visit, see what's up with it then." "Alrighty then, girlfriend. See you in a month" I said, and Avery and I headed for the parking lot.

On my drive home I didn't think much of the lump she felt in my breast or the look of concern on her face. I figured if it was something bad she would have it looked at properly, with an ultrasound or something. She'd have a proper OB/GYN take a look, certainly. So, if she wasn't concerned then neither was I.

So, off we drove to the market to pick up a few things. I had a craving for apples, so we picked up a big bag of my favorite Gala apples, making sure that we chose the best ones to put in the bag. We picked up our other items and headed for home.

We got to the house and Rich was there to help with the groceries. Yay! I headed straight for the bag of apples, picked the prettiest, firmest one I could find and cut right into it. It was the weirdest thing. I cut into this perfectly firm, beautiful apple and it was completely rotten inside. Completely rotten.

I almost dropped the knife when the rotten apple reminded me of a terrible dream I had when I was a kid. A felt like the room was spinning around and around. I managed my way over to the phone to call Julie the Midwife. She answered on the first ring. "Julie? About waiting to check on that lump in my breast in a month? That's not going to work. I need you to make an appointment for me with and OB/GYN today. I have a really bad feeling about this."

CHAPTER 5

One Bad Apple

I've been very lucky with my dream life. I can count the bad dreams I've had in my life on both hands. Don't know why I've been so fortunate, I'm just grateful for it. I have friends who are not so fortunate. I have one friend in particular who is plagued by bad dreams on an almost nightly basis. It is impossible for me to understand why a person whose life is full of kindness and compassion is burdened with nights full of terror and distress. Never has made sense to me and I don't imagine that it ever will. I, on the other hand, have been blessed with a dreamtime full of goodness and comforting thoughts. Well, there is one glaring exception.

When I was about 11 years old and living in my parent's house, I had a doozie of a nightmare. I was sleeping in my white canopy bed that my mom had bought for me. Mine was a room fit for a princess, full of everything that an 11 year old girl could dream up. It was sweet and innocent and full of toys and baby dolls and over-stuffed plush animals. The bed was feminine and beautiful, "Just like you are, Robin-Egg," my mom would say. This was a most unlikely setting for the nightmare I had that night so long ago. In my dream, I sat up in my bed and, from out of the darkness came some reptilian-type monster with huge claws. This "THING" came at me and ripped my nightgown open from top to bottom in one swipe. Then this monster started clawing away at my left breast, ripping and tearing the flesh with his sharp claws. I couldn't move. I couldn't scream. All I could do was look down at this demon shredding my flesh with that evil claw. When the attack stopped I looked down at my breast and it looked just like a rotten apple inside. It was brown and bruised looking, just like a nasty old piece of fruit. Smelled like one, too. Never could make sense of that one.

Why did I at 11 years old have such an evil and violent dream, and why did it seem so real? It felt more like an encounter with some evil being than it did a nightmare. The thought of that dream stayed with me my whole life, drifting into my conscious thoughts from time to time, always wondering why on earth I would have such a dream. I never did think I'd make sense of that one. But one day I did.

After baby Avery and I returned home from our visit with Julie the Midwife and went in to the kitchen to make ourselves a snack, the nightmare that I had had so many years before came back to me like a sick, slow wave. I held in my left hand a healthy, firm, bright red apple, not a bruise on it anywhere. The perfect specimen. Then I placed it on the cutting board, took my favorite fruit knife, sliced it in half and there it was, lying right in front of me on the counter. The rotten apple. It was the apple of my nightmare, I was just sure of it! I grabbed the phone and called Julie the Midwife and I told her to make an appointment for me THAT DAY to have the lump in my breast examined. The perfectly firm, beautiful apple that was rotten inside took me right back to the feeling of that nightmare I had had as a child.... It was all just too weird. So Julie the Midwife made that appointment for me for that very day, and baby Avery and I left that rotten apple on the cutting board, grabbed our stuff and headed off to the hospital. I had no idea at that moment that a new journey was beginning for me and my family. I was just driving to the hospital to have a lump in my breast examined by a professional. Who knew that I was driving right into the middle of a dark and dangerous storm? Who knew that once I drove into this storm, neither I nor anyone who knew me would ever be the same again.

◻ ◻ ◻

I arrived at the hospital with a heaviness in the pit of my stomach, baby Avery in tow. We went straight to the imaging wing and were ushered immediately into the ultrasound room. I was told by the lab technician to undress from the waist up, to put on a hospital gown and to lie down on the examining table. Baby Avery was fascinated by everything in the room and was very curious as to why mommy was lying half naked on a table and some strange woman was rubbing a funny looking stick with a ball on the end of it over her mommy's bosom (or babem, as she called it!). The exam room was dark and quiet, the only sound was the hum of the equipment and the beeping and typing of the ultrasound technician as she carried out her task. She squirted the cold KY Jelly onto my left breast and went to work, looking at the monitor more than the breast, seeing things that only trained professionals can see. As a mother, I'd had plenty of ultrasounds. All new mothers look forward to them. They are joyful occasions when you get to peek in to the very center of yourself, peer behind the sacred cloth to get a glimpse of the Holy of Holies—the baby in your womb. The experience is pure magic and mysticism as you are somehow able to see the un-see-able. It's even more moving to me than seeing the images of our beautiful Universe sent back to us from the Hubble Telescope because you are seeing the images of your own inner universe, with your baby, your precious gift from God, floating around in it's own personal "Space," weightless and free-floating, nourished and safe, completely supported by the womb surrounding it. Today's ultrasound was no such experience. Quite the contrary, in fact. Today's ultrasound was neither mystical nor magical, but fearful and full of dread.

It felt like the lab technician took an inordinate amount of time on my exam. Baby Avery was no longer happily engaged in the newness of these strange surroundings and wanted her mommy to get off of that table and play with her. Or, more likely, she wanted her mommy's "babem" back for herself and away from this strange lady, so that she could be nursed and comforted like she would be on any ordinary day. But the exam went on and on, and I saw the worried look on the lab technician's face as she imaged and probed and typed her findings into her special computer. Finally, she got up from her chair and excused herself, asking me to stay where I was on the exam table until she returned. At this point, I lifted baby Avery up on the table with me and let her nurse a little from the other breast. I held her and fed her and we cuddled and cooed until the nurse returned. As she entered the room I could see the concern on her face, and I asked her what she saw on the ultrasound. She told me in no uncertain terms that she was not supposed to relay any information whatsoever to a patient, that it was not only against hospital protocol but against the law as well. After her disclaimer, she sat herself down on the examining table with me and baby Avery, still suckling at my breast. "I'm not supposed to do this sort of thing, but, considering…." At that, she trailed off. She took a deep breath through her scrunched-up nose and let it out slowly, then continued, "I could get in a lot of trouble for doing this, but I have to tell you, Robin. This doesn't look good. Doesn't look good at all. I've already called the Oncologist on duty today and he's been told about your situation. He's going to meet us over in the mammography room right now."

◻ ◫ ◻

My situation? What did she mean "my situation"? She told the cancer doctor about my situation? I had a situation? What the hell does that mean? My blood turned to ice water and the tears began to flow a little. I held them back as best I could so I wouldn't scare my baby. I didn't want to let on that anything was wrong. Not yet, anyway. So, I scooped up baby Avery and all of our gear and followed the lab technician down a few hallways, through a few wide, swinging hospital doors and in to the mammography waiting room. I sat down, my mind whirling and spinning, trying to hold back the tears. "Wait to worry" I told myself. "Just wait to worry, Robin. Get it together, girl. You don't know anything yet. Just take a deep breath. Find the Zen. Find the Zen…."

Almost immediately the mammography tech came in to the waiting room and motioned for me to go into the exam room. I stood up and moved toward the door with baby Avery coming right behind me. The tech said, " I'm afraid she's going to have to stay out here in the waiting room. There's too much radiation involved in a mammogram. It's very dangerous for babies. Don't worry. She'll be all right with the nurse. Anita will take good care of her. It'll only take a minute."

So I went in to the exam room, the tech closed the door behind me, and baby Avery fell completely apart. "Mommy! Mommy! I want my Mommy! Where IS Mommy? I WANT MY MOMMY!" She wailed and cried and screamed so loud that I thought my heart would break into a million pieces. There was my baby daughter right on the other side of the door screaming for me and there was nothing I could do to comfort her. It was one of the most horrible moments of my life, hearing my baby scream for me and being powerless, absolutely powerless to do anything about it.

The tech ushered me over to the mammogram machine and, as she was arranging my breast on to the cold, hard plastic I asked her if the radiation was dangerous for my baby en utero. She assured me that the special apron she laid over my belly would keep the baby safe. So the exam commenced. She took all the x-rays she needed, from top to bottom, then the side view, the whole time I can hear my baby crying in absolute desperation and confusion and anger from the other side of the door. It was pure torture for both of us. But the exam did finally end, I threw my clothes on as quickly as I could and ran to my baby on the other side of that door and rocked her and soothed her for what seemed like an eternity, until her crying subsided and she felt warm and safe again in her mommy's arms.

Avery and I were told to stay in the waiting room until the Oncologist on duty had a chance to take a look at the x-rays. I have no idea how long we waited. Could have been a minute, could have been an hour. I had no concept of time at the moment, only that Avery was safe in my arms again and with that I was satisfied. The tech came back in to the waiting room and led us to the Oncologists office. The doctor offered us a seat in the chair in front of his huge wooden desk. Behind this desk I could see several x-rays of breasts seen from all angles, presumably mine.

Then he dropped the bomb. "You've got several tumors in your left breast, Mrs. Ellis. One of them is particularly large. The size and shape of these tumors indicate that they are definitely cancer, but we won't know if they are malignant or not until we can do a biopsy on them. I suggest you make an appointment for a needle biopsy today, if possible. Sorry to be the bearer of bad news, Mrs. Ellis, but we better take action on this right away." At that point he gave me the name and number of the best cancer surgeon in the Taos area, shook my hand and, with a very grave and almost apologetic look in his eyes, walked us to the door and said goodbye.

Avery and I walked out of the Hospital and found our car. I put baby Avery in her little car seat with her little eyes still red and puffy from her terrifying experience in the mammography waiting room. I put the key in the ignition, put the car in drive and drove right over to the building site where I knew my husband was working that day. I pulled up to the site, turned the car off and left Avery in her car seat sleeping. I motioned to a couple of the guys to find Rich, and he came walking over toward me. I looked right into his beautiful green eyes and said, "Honey, we're in trouble. We're in a lot of trouble." And with that, I collapsed into his arms, dropped to my knees—unable to stand—incapacitated and unable to breathe, my lungs otherwise occupied with my long, drawn out, soundless sobs that I thought would never end.

CHAPTER 6

Doctor Cetrulo's Shoes

It's difficult to communicate the feeling that you get when you hear your name and the word cancer used in the same sentence. But there it was. I had cancer. The doctor had just said so. "You have several tumors in your left breast, Mrs. Ellis..... and they are definitely cancerous" he had said. And then the world stops for a moment and your body feels heavy like it's filled with quickly hardening concrete. The air around you feels thick somehow, like it's weighing down on you. I just stood there for a moment in a mixture of disbelief and fury. "I have cancer???? What do you mean I have cancer...? I CAN'T have cancer. I'm having a baby, for God's sake!" Of all the feelings swirling around in my mind and body at that moment, fear was the most prominent. I was totally terrified. Was I going to die now? What was going to happen to the baby inside of me? Will baby Avery be left without a mommy? Will Rich have to raise our child alone? So many questions whirling around me all at the same time. I felt intoxicated by it all. But somehow, after that dreadful diagnosis, I found the strength and the wherewithal to gather up my baby, find my car and drive into the day. Outside the hospital walls and outside of my thoughts it was a day like any other. For my family and me, it was the beginning of a journey into the unknown. This was the turning point of my life, of my family's life. This was the day that re-shaped and re-configured life as I knew it before. And it was, from that point on, forever changed.

☐ ☒ ☐

Life around me went along normally in the days that followed my initial diagnosis. The magpies squawked up in the trees, cars drove by with their music blaring on the street in front of our house, the sun came up in the east and set in the west. Everything was as it had always been. But not me. My life did not go along normally in the days and weeks after my preliminary cancer diagnosis. My life was now on hold, in a sense. My mind was consumed with this cancer thing. I couldn't make plans for travel or to entertain friends, couldn't make airline reservations to go visit my parents or anything else, for that matter. All I could do was be still and wait to take the next step on the Cancer Path. The next step for me was a Needle Biopsy. With a Needle Biopsy they could definitively tell whether or not these tumors were cancerous , or so they said. So that was the next step. That was the big plan for my immediate future. Not a fun plan, to be sure. But at least it was a plan. So I made the appointment for the needle biopsy and waited for the day to arrive.

Well, a needle biopsy is just about as much fun as it sounds like it is! (If you've had one you know what I'm talking about!) But, at this point on the Cancer Path, you just take the next step. You do what they tell you to do. You're still in the discovery phase at this point. The "procedures," as they're so fond of calling them, are simple and straightforward and not in any way dangerous for me or my unborn baby. We're just trying to figure out what the heck is going on. So, when the day arrived to go back to the hospital for the "procedure," I went willingly. I had learned enough at this point not to take my toddler with me to the hospital anymore. No more trauma in the waiting room, thank you very much. The biopsy smarted a bit, I must admit. But for me it was more claustrophobic than it was painful, really. They use a device not unlike a mammogram machine whereas it squished your bosom up from the bottom and down from the top until you're as flat as an iHop pancake. Then, as you remain completely motionless, they poke a needle into you and bring out a tissue sample from the tumor itself. The hard part is getting that little bitty needle directly into the tumor. A bit like "Pin the tail IN the Donkey," now that I think about it. So, you have to remain perfectly still while they're pushing this rather wide needle poking out of a huge syringe into a very delicate part of your anatomy! Easy it was not. I was glad when it was over, to be sure. They had a bit of my tumor up and out of my body now. All that was left to do was to wait for the results to come back. All we could do was sit and wait.

You know, in retrospect, waiting for Pathology results was one of the hardest parts of the whole cancer experience for me. Just sitting around waiting for that damn phone to ring. Lord, the endless conversations I had with myself and with God. While we waited, I dusted off some of my old self-help books and went to work on some SERIOUS positive thinking. I used positive affirmations like a Buddhist would use a chant, saying things like, "I am healthy and whole" and "My body is free of disease and full of love and light" over and over again. But, strangely enough, when I'd pray, when I'd actually talk to God, I'd say "Thy will be done," and I'd ask for peace and nothing more. And when I prayed those words to God a funny feeling would come over me sometimes. I would feel calm and still and I just knew that God had it in His hands. I didn't know what the result was going to be, if I was going to live or die, if my baby was going to be stillborn or horribly deformed or if my husband was going to be left behind a widower and single father. I knew NOTHING of my future, (if I even HAD one) or what God had in store for me. But somehow, in certain holy moments, a sense of trust and wellbeing would envelop me and I knew everything was as it was supposed to be. I wish I could say that I felt that every day, but that would be untrue. Truth be told, some days, when the peace would elude me, I just kind of ran around like my hair was on fire. Emotionally speaking, that is.

◌ ▣ ◌

Well, that call finally came. The results were in from the Needle Biopsy. The tumors were, indeed, Cancerous. I took a deep breath and sat down with Rich. We held each other tightly and I soaked his sweatshirt with yet more of my tears. Then we pushed back from one another, sat down at the dining room table and made the call. It was time to schedule an appointment with the surgeon.

Dr. Cetrulo had come highly recommended by all our doctor friends. If you needed to be cut on, he was your man. So we went to see him in his office in Taos. He was friendly and calm, gave us a sense that everything was going to be all right. I felt an instant friendship with Dr. Cetrulo. He was a kind man and could somehow get you laughing when your whole world was falling apart in front of you and you were scared to death. He did a breast exam in his office, took a look at the x-rays and we agreed on the date for the surgery. He explained the "procedure" to us using all the proper medical terminology. All I came away with from that meeting was that he was going to relieve me of a good bit of my left breast. A boob-ectomy, if you will. Well, a PARTIAL boob-ectomy anyway. Oh Lord.... He assured me that he would take as little tissue as was necessary to remove all of the tumors. Tissue? This is my breast we're talking about here! I may not have much in that area, but I've grown very fond of them over the years and I'm not all that excited about having one of them cut into and removed! Yikes! But this was the next step on this Cancer Path, the next phase of the discovery process. They had to get in there and get those tumors out of me and see if they were malignant. Like it or not, they had to remove those tumors, and a good bit of my breast in the process.

The idea of the surgery was a little disconcerting to me, I must admit. And, because I was pregnant, I was going to be wide awake during the whole thing. They gave me a low dosage anti-anxiety pill to take just before the surgery and that, my friends, was that. In the days leading up to the surgery I experienced a mixture of fear of the pain and hope that the tumors they removed from my body would be benign and that this whole chapter in my life could be over and done with forever. Surely, I thought, these tumors couldn't be malignant. I mean, I'm 36 years old! I can't have malignant tumors in my breast, right? Nah, they were going to be benign, I just KNEW it. So, off to the surgery we went.

I took my little anti-anxiety pill on the way to the hospital, but I can't say it helped me very much. I was terrified. I'd never had any type of surgery before in my life, and for my "maiden voyage," if you will, I had to be wide awake! Well, we got to the hospital and they got me into my hospital gown, put me on the gurney and away we went to the operating room. There were so many people in the room! I couldn't figure out why they were all there. Dr. Cetrulo and I were cracking jokes with each other (my way of dealing with my fear, I guess), and then it was time. They put up what they called a tent, which disabled me from being able to see them perform the surgery.

This "tent" was basically a small sheet that spanned the short distance from my left shoulder and collar bone up toward the left side of my face. They used a numbing drug shot directly into my breast area with a syringe, gave it a minute or two to take effect, and away he went. I could see Dr. Cetrulo's face and the faces of the surgical staff standing around me. They all looked so serious. Well, I guess that's a GOOD thing, now that I think about it! You don't want your surgeon and his staff standing around telling funny stories or recalling tales of botched operations they'd heard about or anything like that! A serious demeanor was appropriate, to be sure. Dr. Cetrulo looked me in the eye and asked, "Are you ready, Robin?"

"Let's do this thing," I responded. And with that, Dr. C began the "procedure."

It was a curious feeling, having surgery while I was wide awake. The sensation that I remember the most was the feeling of having my skin spread apart, like if you take your fingers from your right hand and put them on your left forearm all in a clump and then spread the fingers apart from each other while applying pressure. A feeling of pulling and stretching the skin of my breast apart, pushing it apart, one side from the other. Strange sensation to say the least. I felt no pain, just that strange pulling sensation. All I could do was look into the faces of Dr. C and his staff all standing around me. Those folks have mastered their poker faces --- I could read nothing in their eyes. After the doctor removed the tumors and the tissue surrounding them, he sewed up the wound on what was left of my breast and they wheeled me off to the recovery room.

Rich was waiting for me there. It was so good to see his face and feel his love and support. The recovery room was small and dark. Felt like we were in a hospital broom closet or something. I was relieved that the surgery was over and terrified about what we were going to find out today. I had begged Dr. C to not make us wait for the pathology results, having explained to him that another week of sitting by the phone NOT KNOWING would have been unbearable. Well, today we didn't have to wait for our results. Dr. Cetrulo pulled some strings for us that day. He had rushed the breast tissue up to the lab and gotten the results before I was even out of the recovery room. When he came in to meet us in that small, dark room, he didn't have to say a word. We could read it on his face. But he did speak. "It's bad, guys…. It's a bad one…. I'm so sorry…," he said, and you could tell that he was genuinely sad about it, too.

Me, I was shocked and more than a little mad. I was crying out of anger and frustration and fear, asking the doctor, "well what do we do now? How bad is it? What do you mean 'it's a bad one'?"

He told us right then and there that we'd need another surgery to take out more of the tissue surrounding the tumors, and that they'd have to remove the lymph nodes in the pit of my left arm. "And the sooner the better, guys. We'd better see exactly what we're dealing with here. Call my office later this afternoon and we'll find the next possible day for your surgery. I'm truly sorry, guys. I was hoping to have some good news for you today." And with that he left Rich and me on our own in the recovery room, totally in shock. And then, as if to add insult to injury, the local anesthetic they had used on me during the surgery began to wear off, and the pain started to get my attention. Pain has a way of doing that, doesn't it.

◻ ◻ ◻

Wow. Wow wow wow. I mean just simply WOW! I had CANCER! The real deal! The most dreaded words in the English language, (or ANY language, for that matter!), and I had just heard them. "It's a bad one!," Dr. Cetrulo had said. A bad one. That meant malignant. I guess I'd earned the right to use the actual word by now. I had a tumor and it was MALIGNANT. Great. Just great…… And now I have another surgery scheduled in six days. SIX DAYS, for God's sake! The pain had set in and it was substantial, to be sure. I just tried to keep my mind off of the next surgery and what they might find then. It had been nothing but bad news so far, so why should the next surgery be any different???? I felt so defeated in those days. I felt angry and resentful, I just wasn't sure at what or at whom. I had had SUCH a blessed life up until then. Born into money and privilege, adored by my parents, popular and attractive, not a door I'd ever run into that I couldn't open. I was the type that could always talk my way into or out of any situation—but not this one. I wanted to demand to "speak to the manager" or "customer service" or SOMEONE who could fix this problem for me. I was plagued by this, "Don't you know who I am?" mentality. I don't know if it looked as pathetic as it felt, but this was brand new territory for me and I had NO IDEA how to deal with it. What I DID know was that there was no way to wiggle out of this one, and that made me madder than anything. Inside I felt like a 2 year old who hadn't gotten her way and I wanted to lie down on the floor and throw a major hissy fit! There's no getting around this one, though. No one you can talk to. No one who can just "make it go away." Your husband can't "love it away' and your parents can't bail you out of it and your doctor can't write you a note to excuse you from it. You are IN IT, and NO ONE CAN RESCUE YOU AND MAKE IT ALL GO AWAY…. Well, there's a first time for everything, I guess. And, I must admit, I didn't like it ONE LITTLE BIT!

◙ ◙ ◙

So, the day arrived for the second surgery. Rich was there with me as was my girlfriend Jenny Bird. I think they were there to support each other as much as to support me. For this surgery, Dr. Cetrulo and his team had decided to put me to sleep with as little anesthesia as possible so as to not adversely affect my baby en utero. They decided this, they told us, because they were going to have to cut me open AGAIN in the same area they had cut into only six days before, which was already in a lot of pain. And, they told us, that the underarm area where they had to operate to retrieve the lymph nodes was very sensitive. So, the decision was made. This particular surgery I was to sleep through. So I'm back in the same hospital, in the same hospital gown, in the same operating room with the same faces surrounding me. Then one of them put a mask over my nose and mouth and told me to count backwards from 100. I think I made it to about 99, and I was O-U-T out!

I woke up in another recovery room than the one before. This one was brightly lit with several other patients lined up beside me, also recovering from various surgeries. When I opened my eyes I saw Rich and Jenny Bird standing over me, asking me if I was ok, and did I need anything. I tried to sit up a bit, and then the pain hit me. I had the most intense stinging sensation under my arm and an awful deep throbbing pain in my left breast.

I wanted to crawl right out of my body, right out of the pain. I could barely stand it! I kept sitting up higher and higher on the gurney, literally trying to get away from the pain. But, of course, I couldn't. I couldn't BELIEVE how much it hurt! I had never experienced pain like that before in my life, and I had just been through natural childbirth! I had nothing to compare it to. I didn't think I'd make it without screaming out.

At that very moment, Dr. Cetrulo pushed back the curtain and poked his head into the room. He read the pain and anguish on my face and motioned to the nurse to come and give me a little bit more morphine. As the nurse was administering the morphine into my IV and I was beginning to relax just a little bit, Dr. Cetrulo said it again….. "It's a bad one, kids. I'm so sorry to have to tell you this, but 17 of the 22 lymph nodes are malignant. I'm afraid the Cancer has metastasized." With that information swimming around in my head, I sat straight up, looked at him directly in the eyes, and threw up all over Dr. Cetrulo's shoes.

CHAPTER 7

Jenny Grabs a Broom

The pain after my second surgery was ridiculous. It took me almost a week before I could function normally in my world again. My family and friends and I had decided that I should plan some recovery time somewhere besides my own home. Avery was a year and a half old and certainly could not understand what was wrong with Mommy and why she couldn't play with her. I just couldn't bear the thought of being debilitated in front of my baby and the confusion and pain that it would undoubtedly cause her, so we decided on an alternate plan. In the six days between the first and second surgeries I was home with baby Avery and we were playing together outside.

One of her favorite things to do was for me to grab both of her arms and swing her around and around like a helicopter. She begged me and begged me to play Helicopter with her, and I just didn't have the heart to say no. So I grabbed her arms and swung her up in the air. We swung around and around and she laughed and laughed and then I slowed us down a bit until she came to a landing back on the ground again. "More Mommy! Again, again!" she kept crying. I wanted so badly to play our fun game, the one she loved so much, the one that gave her such joy. But I felt the pain and looked down at my shirt and there was blood seeping through from my surgery wound, and we had to stop. She was sad but easily distracted, so we found something else we could do together that didn't make Mommy bleed. After that rather depressing revelation, we booked a hotel room for me and two of my girlfriends for a few days after my second surgery while I regained my strength and gave the pain some time to subside. And Rich, my precious Rich, stayed home and took care of our Avery.

You know, now that I think about it, Rich did AN AWFUL LOT of things that were above and beyond the call of duty while all of this was going on. You see, cancer doesn't just happen to one person. It happens to everyone around them, too. The only difference is that when you are the one who is sick, you have folks around you telling you how to fight it, how to beat it, how to tackle this thing and (hopefully) get better. You're on the Cancer Path now! You start at "A" and you end at "Z" and hopefully, when it's all said and done, you're alive to tell the tale. Cancer becomes who you are and what you do, kind of like a coat that you put on or a club that you join. I'm in the Cancer Club now! That's how it feels!

You begin to identify yourself by your disease. There is a sort of belonging that is hard to put into words. It's kind of like when you have kids. When you're wheeling your baby around in her stroller at the park or at the mall and you make eye contact with another mother, there is a silent exchange of information that moves between you, a secret that you both share that only mothers fully understand. It's unspoken yet completely understood. It's like that for cancer patients, too, in a way. But for the ones who love the cancer patient, the friends and the family and the neighbors and the co-workers, even your casual friends and acquaintances—there is no protocol on how to act, no books written on the subject (to the best of my knowledge) and no one, I mean NO ONE knows what to do.

Cancer is a very selfish disease. This may be true of other life-threatening diseases, too, I don't know. But I DO know that Cancer is spectacularly selfish. I was completely self-consumed during this time in my life. My husband described it as me being "out of my body" for the duration of the treatment, and for years afterward, too. I went deep into a world of my own, slipped further and further inside of myself, and basically let everything around me take care of itself. I was incapable of performing the day to day tasks of normal life. I found it very difficult to clean the house, make the beds, feed the family, interact with my child, or even answer the telephone.

I came to rely greatly on our electronic devices, like answering machines and computers. I found talking on the phone excruciatingly difficult, so I'd let our machine pick up all our calls. I found that e-mail was much, much easier and less threatening, so I did most of my correspondence through the computer. I was like a remote and lonely island, cut off and disconnected from the water that surrounded it. I was oblivious and unreachable. I was quiet and introspective. I was totally unlike my normal, healthy self, and this fact, I believe, was as difficult for my friends and family to deal with as was the cancer itself. I'm totally convinced that cancer is more difficult for family and loved ones than it is for the person who is actually sick. Strange, I know, but undeniably true. In retrospect I have a greater understanding of what my family and friends went through during our journey, (because it was, indeed, OUR journey!) but only because I asked. Took me years to ask, but I asked. "What was it like when I was sick? What was I like? What was it like for you?"

Like I said, it took me YEARS to ask. It took that long for the selfishness of it all to wear off enough to even REALIZE how heavy it was for everyone who loved me. It took me a while to realize how much time I had lost with Avery and Rich, and took me even longer to come to terms with the fact that I was TOTALLY disconnected from the baby in my womb. I was afraid to connect with my unborn baby—petrified that she might die or be horribly impaired—scared to connect with this little soul that I may very well never get the chance to know or to love. I was horrified at the prospect that my saving myself might in fact be killing the child inside of me. I just couldn't go there. The intensity of it all completely overwhelmed me, and I just "checked out," disconnected my self. Esoterically speaking, I tucked tail and ran deep inside myself to some secret place I'd found that felt safe. That secret place where the soul lives. That's where I needed to go.... And that's where I needed to stay....

I was one of the very lucky ones, though. Yes, I was burdened with a life-threatening disease, didn't know if I or my baby would live or die, I looked like a freak, I was tired and sick and had half a boob, but I still consider myself one of the very lucky ones. I had an amazing support system around me that made my life function. Without them I don't know how I would have made it through. And every one of my family and close friends handled the cancer in a completely different way. Their ways of coping were as unique and different as they are. But it all added up to a perfect little support system, everyone doing something totally different to help and support me and my family through this nightmare. And for that I am deeply grateful.

◻ ▣ ◻

Well, now it was time to take the next step on the Cancer Path. It was time to meet the Cancer Doctor. I even learned the name for cancer doctors which was a word that was not previously in my vocabulary: Oncologist. Oh great, now it's time to meet our Oncologist. The word sounds so sinister, doesn't it? Anyway, this was the next step on the Path, so we made all the necessary inquiries and found an oncologist in Santa Fe, and we made the preliminary appointment with him and our surgeon, all of us to meet together at the same place at the same time. It was time to map out our plan of attack.

Meeting Dr. Lopez for the first time was not the happiest of occasions. He's a great guy, don't get me wrong, and he came highly recommended. It's just a tough day when you and your husband have to sit in a doctor's office at the New Mexico Cancer Care Center to discuss whether or not they're going to be able to save you and your baby's life or not. "What are the odds, doc? We'd really love to know."

Well, we had much to discuss, and discuss we did. All things considered, Dr. Lopez and Dr. Cetrulo had three main options for us to choose from. But first, the facts. I had stage 2 Breast Cancer, so far as they KNEW. They couldn't do an MRI or x-rays to see if there were more tumors in any other organs. X-rays are, of course, too dangerous for my baby en utero. So, here were their treatment options: a) terminate my pregnancy before starting chemo (this one was TOTALLY out of the question, so we moved on to: b) withhold chemo treatment until after the baby is born (which, we found out, is almost certain death for me because breast cancer is fueled by estrogen and progesterone and we all know how much of THAT is swimming around a pregnant woman's body, so we moved on to c) begin chemo treatment DURING pregnancy, starting at the beginning of the 3rd trimester…. "I'm sorry, Doc, can you just repeat that last option one more time? I thought I heard you say that we were going to start chemotherapy while the baby is still inside of me!"

"There is very little research on this particular medical situation, Robin, but I can sum up what we've found in our research."

"Yeah, I really wish you would!"

Then our oncologist and our surgeon agreed, and voiced what they'd learned. "If you terminate the pregnancy, we can move along with treatment immediately and normally. But, since you and Rich are vehemently opposed to that, we'll move on to our other options. In the few studies we could find, the women that we've read about who've refused treatment until their baby was born have all passed away. Bar none. On the other hand, the cases that we've studied of women who have received chemotherapy while still pregnant, so long as they begin during their third trimester, reports have been very positive for both mother and baby. There was only one report of a baby who had been subject to chemotherapy en utero who turned out to be autistic, but, because of the mother's age and medical background the child had a high risk of autism anyway, so that they don't think it was caused in any way by the chemotherapy."

That last sentence I paid no attention to. It sounded like when the grown ups talk on the "Peanuts" cartoons—bwah bwah bwah bwah bhaw. I was in TOTAL shock....."Now, let me get this straight.... Now you guys are trying to tell me that because I'm pregnant, I can't drink and I can't smoke cigarettes and I should stay away from salty foods, but that CHEMOTHERAPY IS OK????????? What are you CRAZY?????" We were completely dumbfounded. They were completely serious. They wanted to start chemotherapy right away because of the grave nature of the cancer and how quickly it was spreading through my body, but, they decided, it was more prudent to wait until I was in the 3rd trimester of my pregnancy. That very day, if possible.

So we left the meeting completely speechless. We had a LOT of decisions to make. Now it was time to decide who to trust and what path we were going to take. We didn't like our choices very much, but they're the only ones we had. Terminate the pregnancy? No way. Wait to start treatment until the baby is born and risk the baby having no mommy? Doesn't sound so good. Start chemotherapy with a baby inside of me?

Unthinkable! We had some serious soul searching to do. And it had be done as soon as possible.

◻ ◻ ◻

We had to make a decision, and we had to make if fast. We began doing our own research on the Web, trying to find as much information as we could on pregnant women and breast cancer. We could find almost NONE! Our doctors were correct when they had told us that very little research had been done and there were very few reports of ANY women in the United States who had been affected by this or about what they had done about it. All we could find were reports of women who had been diagnosed with breast cancer during pregnancy, had refused treatment and who had perished shortly after their child was born. We found a few accounts of women in the same situation who had decided on chemotherapy DURING pregnancy, and they and their babies were fine. There were no further studies done on those babies as they grew up, though. Were there learning disabilities? Were there any emotional or physical problems down the line? No one knew. It was all a big secret. No one, not even the Medical Establishment of the United States of America could tell us exactly what was going to happen to our baby if we decided to start treatment with our baby still en utero. It was all one big, terrifying mystery.

◻ ◻ ◻

Our household was very solemn to say the least. Rich and I studied what research we could get our hands on, talked to every doctor we knew and worked furiously to try to come up with our own plan. We weighed the risks against the benefits over and over again. We cried a lot. We prayed constantly. And then we decided. We decided to trust our doctors, to put my life and the life of our unborn child in their care. The decision was made. We would start chemotherapy on the very first day of the third trimester of my pregnancy. So there it was. This was the moment. We were ready to surrender.

In the weeks that followed, we waited for 'the big day' in something that looked and felt like a coma. We walked and we talked but it was as if we were sleepwalking. Our family would check in on us daily, offering their love and support. Our friends would call from time to time and do the same. There were casseroles dropped by for us and pies and cakes delivered from our friends who lived nearby, everyone trying to relieve the stress from our everyday lives, but not really knowing how. And then there was Jenny. Jenny dropped by one day without calling first during the "sleepwalking" period, while we were waiting for our own personal "D-Day" to arrive. She walked in the door, gave me a quick kiss on the cheek, gave baby Avery a big squeeze, and, without saying a word, Jenny grabbed a broom and started sweeping. By the time she left, our entire house was clean. Then she pecked me on the cheek again, whisked out the door without saying a word, and left. She didn't say anything, she just grabbed a broom. Just grabbed that broom and started cleaning.... I had no idea how much I needed someone to do JUST that. Nothing more. Nothing less. Just grab a broom.

CHAPTER 8

The Healing Ceremony

Well, our decision had been made. We were going to do the unthinkable. We were going to begin my chemotherapy while my baby was still inside of me. It's hard, if not impossible to describe how I felt having made that decision. We had weighed out our options and had looked at the facts and we had studied all the reports that we could get our hands on. And then we prayed. We put our lives and the life of our unborn baby in God's hands. We felt certain that we were doing the right thing for everyone concerned— but we were still sick with worry over our unborn baby. We trusted God completely, that whatever He had in store for us was for our highest good. But that didn't relieve our worry of what was to come. We weren't sure we could handle what was in front of us, even if it was God's will. We knew we were in His hands, yet still we were not comforted.

We had made the move from Taos to Santa Fe for the simple fact that I needed anonymity. Rich completely understood my need to 'disappear', and he moved our household in a single day. We were very fortunate that his family owned a three-house compound in the Arroyo Hondo neighborhood of Santa Fe, and we made camp in one of them. The house was big and private and empty, but as we moved our belongings into the stone house it felt more and more like home. Rich and Avery and I shared one big bedroom, and through time we made it our own.

Looking back over the timeline of my Cancer Journey, I wonder how we got through it all. We found out we were pregnant with our second child in October of 2000, when Avery was not yet 1 year old. Julie the Midwife found the lump in my breast two months later. The two surgeries and the discovery of the cancer was in January of 2001, and yet treatment didn't begin until April of the same year. We had to wait three whole months to start treatment after the diagnosis. We had to wait until I was in my third trimester. The doctors had deemed it imperative. We couldn't figure out for the life of us what difference it would make to wait, but the doctors had explained that once the baby was in the third trimester, all of their little body parts and their major organs were fully formed. In the third and final trimester of pregnancy the babies just got bigger and stronger and better prepared to face the world outside of the womb. And so, once again, we decided to trust our doctors. And thus began the waiting.

◌ ◌ ◌

So, we were waiting for D-Day. My first chemo treatment was scheduled for April 3 and it was only February, the dreariest month of all in New Mexico, and all we could do was wait. Day to day life began to take shape in our new home. I was still in my oblivion, but I remember bits and pieces of those waiting months. I was, as always, unable to deal with the mundane chores and responsibilities of tending to house and family, so I drifted through the house day after day, half inside of my body, half outside of it. I remember the feelings of longing and guilt running side by side one another. I longed to be a part of normal life—to cook meals in our new kitchen and play games with my beautiful baby girl, but I could do none of it. It was all I could do to get out of bed in the morning. The fear and the unknowing was debilitating. Life continued around me, but I was not a part of it.

My parents, God bless them, had hired full time help for us, so all I had to do was zombie around the house, really. Rich kept himself busy, and Avery just kept being Avery, toddling around with her sweet yellow hair falling around her face and framing the most beautiful blue eyes I'd ever seen. She, of course, knew nothing of what was going on around her. I mean, how could she, right? She was just a little peanut, couldn't even talk yet except to say "mommy" and "daddy" and "bird" and "babem." She couldn't even pronounce her name yet—called her self Wee Wee Toe, her sweet version of Avery Nicole. All she wanted to do was play and be comforted like any little girl of her age. There was a beautiful, weeping bush outside in the courtyard of the house which made a perfect little fort for her. Avery would sit underneath its boughs and play with her little toys and doo dads and the gravel on the ground. A few times I was able to muster up the strength to sit under there with her. The light came in a lovely, light green color as the sun shone through the leaves, and it felt safe in there somehow. We would sit under there playing with her little dolls and toys, speaking the secret language of mother and baby with one another and I would forget, for a moment, why we were there in that foreign place instead of in our home in Taos, visiting with friends, going to our mother's group in the park and living our normal life.

I wondered during that time if my tiny toddler daughter had some concept of what was happening to her mommy, what a grave and uncertain future I battled with inside of my head. I wondered if she knew of the pain I still felt from the surgeries or of the fear that constantly consumed me. Could she know, I wondered? Could she possibly conceive of such complex concepts as these? But I would pass the thought off as a whim, and once again I could stare into my daughter's beautiful eyes and think nothing of the time past or the time to come. There, under the weeping bush in the courtyard of our Santa Fe house with my daughter, I could find solace. There, for a moment at least, I found peace.

◻ ◻ ◻

There were a few projects to keep us busy during the waiting months, and I was very grateful for the diversion. We had decided to fashion a recovery room, of sorts, out of one of the bedrooms in the house. We had deemed it the "Chemo Room." We figured it would be a good idea if I had a private space of my own to convalesce once my chemo treatments had begun. No one knows exactly how chemotherapy will affect them—some have very little side effects from it while others are completely debilitated by nausea and fatigue. Just in case I fell into the latter category, we thought we had better be prepared. It's terrifying for a child to see a parent seriously ill, and we wanted to spare our Avery that agony. So, the "Chemo Room" came into being. We dressed the bed up as comfy and as pretty as we could, made it nice and dark, put in a little stereo system ready with a big stack of "Relaxation" CD's and installed a TV and VCR, too, with a tall stack of videos next to it. We thought that laughter would be a good tonic, so we brought in all of my favorite comedies and "Chick Movies," as Rich liked to call them.

Once our "Chemo Room" project was complete, we traveled in another direction entirely. We began looking for loopholes along the Cancer Path, thinking that perhaps, just perhaps, we might find a way to lessen our unborn baby's exposure to the harsh and deadly chemicals in the chemotherapy drugs. We thought if we could induce her labor early, get her out of my womb faster, it would reduce her exposure to the Chemo and, perhaps, give her a better chance for a normal life. When we started down this pioneer path we decided it would be prudent to tour the "Preemie" ward at the hospital. We wanted to see for ourselves what these babies looked like—at one month premature, 6 weeks, 8 weeks, and even earlier.

It didn't take us long to make up our minds once we had toured the Intensive Care Unit for Premature Babies. We would do what our doctors had told us; leave the baby in the womb for as long as possible. The babies that don't get baked long enough inside of their mother's womb have a tough time of it. Their little lungs can't work on their own, so they're all hooked up to respirators. All manner of wires connected to an endless array of wildly beeping monitors and machines that these little premature babies were tethered to. It looked so unnatural in there, like those babies weren't supposed to be there yet. Well, in essence they weren't!

But God had a plan for these little critters, apparently, because they were hanging on to life on the thinnest little thread I've ever seen. Many of them made it, we heard later. Some, of course, did not. But weighing the odds of our unborn baby being exposed to the chemo drugs and trusting that the placenta would protect her inside of my womb against the idea of inducing labor and taking her out early—believe it or not, it was an easy call. So, we put aside our pioneer project, and went squarely back on to our Cancer Path, feeling confident that we had made the right decision by deciding to surrender to our doctors and their suggestions once again.

We began a relationship with a new group of doctors during this time, the pre-natal specialists. We would visit them once a week and they would do an ultrasound each visit and measure our growing baby inside of my womb. This time around we knew the gender of our baby before it was born. It was another girl, and we decided on her name right away. Our little baby girl, our little "Cancer Baby" would have a beautiful name, indeed. We named her Tess Elizabeth while she was still safe inside of my womb, before she was bombarded by the chemo drugs, before her future became uncertain. Not knowing if she would live or die, not knowing if she would be normal or horribly impaired, we named that baby girl inside of my womb, and we gave her a unique and beautiful name, indeed. A name that we both loved: Tess Elizabeth Ellis. Our baby had a name now, and that made us feel more connected with her than ever before. We were having a little girl, and our little girl had a name. She was SOMEBODY now, a real human being. God, how we prayed for her safety and well-being. Our knees were black and blue from spending so much time on them praying to God to let her be ok, somehow. "Please spare our little one, God. Please let her be healthy and normal. And please, most of all, let her live."

◘ ◙ ◙

Time passed during the waiting months. Winter turned to spring, and the winds began to blow and blow as they did every year. The sky was the color of turquoise and the hollyhocks began to bloom. It was hard to enjoy the warm sun and the budding flowers as our D-Day was just around the corner. This was the darkest period of all for me, I believe. The waiting months had become the waiting weeks, then the waiting days. I had bad dreams and woke up with the sheets soaked with perspiration. My heart would race during the day as I thought about what was to come. This dark period lifted a bit when my parents came for a visit. My parents, you see, are my very dear friends and the love I have for them is hard to describe, so I won't even try. Just let it be understood that a visit from them made everything seem better. Life was safer somehow when they were around.

One day during their visit, we decided to take baby Avery on a little walk to enjoy the warm sun and all of the bounty of springtime. We applied our sunscreen and donned our hats and set out on a walk on the compound. All three of the Ellis Family houses were connected by a beautiful little gravel path winding through the *pinon* and juniper trees as well as the cactus and the stubby little chamisa bushes. There were ant hills teeming with activity, stink bugs out on their daily march over the desert floor and birds of all descriptions flying around us, squealing and squawking their protests as we got closer and closer to their new spring nests. We ventured up the hill to the big house and marveled at the view of the Sangre de Cristo Mountains. The colors of the High Desert are unique in their subtle hues and soft tones. The mountains were a dark purple resting upon the soft pink dirt of the foreground and capped with the never ending turquoise sky.

Avery led the way for us on our walk, running from one fascinating thing to the next, stomping on the ant hills and playing with the beetles with a stick she had found. She led us all around the gravel path, showing us little treasures all along the way, busy in the way that toddlers always are. Then all of a sudden, she stopped dead in her tracks and she looked back at me. Baby Avery motioned for me to come over to her, and I thought she had found something new and wonderful to show me.

But she had something else on her mind. She grabbed my hand and pulled me down and motioned for me to sit down on the gravel path. I followed her instructions as my mom and dad stood and watched. Then baby Avery came over to me and lifted my shirt up over where my surgery scars were. "Mommy stay," she said, and put her little hand up for me to stop and be still, so I sat there on the gravel path, holding my shirt up, wondering what on earth she had up her sleeve. Then little Avery got busy. She gathered three distinctly different little piles of things she had found and laid them out neatly on the railroad tie at the edge of the path. She reached out with her little hands and gathered up all of the ingredients of the first pile and brought them over to me.

Without saying a word, she took her little hand filled with tiny gravel rocks and rubbed them, ever so gently, over my surgery scars—first over the wound on my bosom, then over the wound under my arm. She rubbed and rubbed, very methodically, silent the entire time. Then she emptied her hands of the gravel, went back to the railroad tie and picked up the second pile of ingredients she had gathered. She brought them over to me and took that tiny hand of hers and rubbed a handful of dried grass and leaves over my wounds. Once again she rubbed and rubbed, ever so gently and very methodically, silent the entire time. Then she emptied her hands of the dried grass and leaves and returned to the railroad tie and picked up the third pile and came back over to me. In her tiny hands she held a handful of new, green leaves which she rubbed and rubbed, ever so gently and very methodically over my wounds, silent the whole time. Then she stood up and, having completed her task, gave me a bright, beautiful little smile, wiped her hands on her shorts and continued on down the little gravel path. I sat there sobbing, my parents standing behind me doing the same.

What had we just witnessed? We were all dumbfounded yet deeply moved by what had just happened. My baby daughter had just performed a Healing Ceremony on me, I was certain of it. We could hardly believe it, though we had just seen it with our own eyes. Where had it come from? How could a baby have knowledge of such things? It was mystical and magical, as if she had channeled some great KNOWING from an unknown source. Was this talent hiding somewhere in her DNA? Did we have a great healer in our ancestral past whose talents were passed down to her through our bloodline? No one will ever know for sure. But there is one thing that I am certain of: that miracles and magic happen every day, even in the midst of a terrible crisis. It's just that some days those miracles are so great that you can't help but notice them. It's just that some days it happens to come from a tiny little being performing a great big miracle with little bitty hands.

CHAPTER 9

Eyes Wide Open

Well before any of us knew about the cancer, before any of us knew about the tumors in my breast and lymph, before any of us knew how much our lives were about to be turned upside down, Jenny Bird had a dream. Now, she didn't tell me about this dream just after she had it because, she said, she didn't want to scare me. The dream, as it turns out, was quite disturbing. She had this dream when I was just barely pregnant, about the time we had found out the news from Julie the Midwife and had almost passed out cold right there on the floor of the Midwifery Center! After we had gotten over the shock and our feelings of overwhelm had turned into excitement and joy we did what every expecting couple does: we called our families, our friends and everyone else we could think of with the great news. We were having another baby! Baby #2 should be born in the summertime—June to be exact. And we shared our joy with anyone who would listen. Even the checkers at the grocery store knew! Pregnancy and baby news is always such a joyful thing and we felt like Santa Claus on Christmas morning with a bag full of presents for everyone. A new baby in a small town is a big deal, and we were celebrating right along side Taos. Our little town was going to have a new baby and everyone, I mean EVERYONE, was just over the moon with excitement.

I could barely wait to call Jenny Bird and tell her the good news, and when I did call her I didn't get the response I expected. What I got was a brief silence on the other end of the line, followed by the usual words of love and congratulations. I didn't think much about the momentary silence until much later—until after I had been diagnosed and she shared her dream with me.

Jenny dreamed I was pregnant, and that she was attending the birth. As I pushed the baby out and brought her up to my breast to feed her, there appeared a circle of thorns around my breast, and the baby couldn't get to it to suckle. In her dream Jenny was worried. How would the baby survive? How would she be able to eat and get strong if Robin's breast was circled by a ring of thorns? At that moment, the baby turned into a little hummingbird, and my nipple turned into a beautiful red rose, and the tiny little hummingbird was able to navigate around the thorns to get to the rose, and that tiny little hummingbird drank and drank of the nectar, and then Jenny knew that the baby was going to be fine. She just turned herself into a little hummingbird and drank from the rose, and she was nourished. The baby would live and thrive. Both mother and baby would be just fine. And with that, the dream ended, and Jenny Bird was comforted.

◘ ◙ ◘

Before our baby could be born, she was exposed to 3 rounds of chemotherapy en utero. We had, of course, researched and dug around for ANY other option, any other course of action that we might take to spare our baby this horrendous and harsh reality inside of the womb, but we could not, with good conscience, come up with a better idea than the one that our doctor's had recommended: leave the baby en utero for as long as possible and hope and pray that the chemotherapy does not adversely affect her. Easy words to say, I know. But it was hell on earth for us, for Rich and me, waiting and wondering, feeling confident in our doctor's expertise and yet terrified that we were harming, even killing our unborn child. We've never prayed so hard in our lives—prayed for our doctors, that they would be Divinely led to make the right decisions; prayed for our baby, that she would be somehow unharmed by the harsh chemicals that were coursing through her body as they were coursing through mine; and prayed for ourselves, that we would remain clear and to know God's will for us—basically we prayed that we were doing the right thing for our unborn baby and that she would be alright. We were praying for a seemingly impossible miracle, and we knew that. But we just kept on and on, hoping beyond hope that SOMEHOW our baby would be healthy and fine, hoping that she would somehow be surrounded by Grace and, against all possible odds, be unharmed.

⚬ ⚬ ⚬

When the day arrived for our baby to be born, I was lying on the Acupuncture table receiving a treatment. My Chinese doctor offered me a needle in a very special point on my foot that day, and I agreed to it. After he had put the needles in all of the usual places on my body—to strengthen my immune system, my liver and other key organs to ward off the negative side affects of chemotherapy—he put a needle in the very special point on my foot, and I felt the tiniest little contraction. My Chinese doctor and I decided that if we were going to have to induce labor in the hospital later that day that we should, if we could, give the baby a little forewarning of what was to come.

I could imagine that babies that are chemically induced are quite surprised and, perhaps unprepared for the birth process they are forced into by the induction drugs. Normally it's the baby itself that releases the hormone into the mother's bloodstream that begins the birthing process. Amazing, isn't it! The baby somehow "knows" when the time is right to be born and initiates the process herself! But when a baby is induced, perhaps it's not, in fact, ready or prepared. It must be a big shock to those babies whose task of initiating the birth process is usurped by the introduction of a very strong chemical from somewhere outside of itself.

Anyway, I felt that after what our baby had been through en utero, perhaps a gentle little nudge toward the birth delivered by an Acupuncture point on my foot might just be the kindest and most humane thing I could do for her. So we did, and the contraction came at the exact moment that he put that needle in my foot. It was amazing, and I knew that I had done a little something to make this day, her birthday, as kind and loving and gentle as I possibly could. It was a tiny act of compassion, but it's all I knew to do. And it did make me feel just a little bit better. And, I'd like to think it helped our baby just a little bit, too.

So, it was time to go to the hospital. The day had arrived to bring our baby into this world and come face to face with The Truth. What

– 59 –

was in store for our baby girl who had withstood so much hardship en utero? Would her body be complete or would she be horribly disfigured? Would she be normal? How could she be? Would she have terrible learning disabilities? Would she even survive the birth? How could a creature so small and helpless overcome such atrocities? How would we ever face her, and how would we ever summon the strength to deal with a lifetime spent coping with a disabled child—one whose disabilities we had caused ourselves? Whatever The Truth was, we were about to come face to face with it, and all the fears and misgivings we had felt in the previous months came flooding over us on this day. The moment had arrived, and we prayed for the strength to handle what was in front of us. All we knew for sure was one thing---- that we would love our baby daughter no matter what. We loved her already. Always had. Always would.

◌ ◌ ◌

Rich and I had placed our little Avery with his sister and had packed up our little bags, one for me and one for baby, and headed off to the big hospital in Albuquerque. Because this birth was "special" we had been instructed to have our baby in the larger, better equipped "big city" hospital— "… Just in case…." the doctors had said. So, off we went to Albuquerque. We were met there by my parents and girlfriends, and we all settled in for the long day (and night!) to come. I had decided on an epidural this time. I mean, why not, right? My situation had forced me into a hospital birth, complete with all the machines tethered to my body and the constant noise emanating from them and every other imaginable institutional irritant. This was not the atmosphere to tough it out with natural childbirth, nor was I strong enough, physically or emotionally, to be able to pull off another birth like we had experienced with our first child.

A few hours after we had arrived, the doctor came in and administered the induction drug into my bloodstream. The clock was ticking now. Shortly afterward, another doctor came in and injected me with the epidural. Rich held me while she put this rather painful and unusual drug directly into my spine, and from then on I had no feeling in my body from the waist down. The epidural made me feel a bit intoxicated and sleepy, so Rich joined my girlfriends, Jenny and Jona, outside on the hospital grounds while I rested. While I laid back and let myself be supported by the bed beneath me, I peered out the window, and a tiny shadow caught my eye. I refocused on the object outside my window, and I suddenly realized what it was. It was a little hummingbird hovering right outside of my hospital window. Sure as I was lying on that bed, there in front of me, just on the other side of the window glass, was a beautiful little hummingbird. I burst into tears at the sight of it. I laid there in that hospital bed, numb from the waist down, donning my little pink cap to cover up my bald head and cried like the baby I was about to give birth to. It was just too much to fathom, too much to take in all at once. As I lay there, crying and pondering this mini-miracle, Rich and the girls burst into the room and said, "Did you see it? Did you see it? There was a…." "HUMMINGBIRD OUTSIDE THE WINDOW!" we all said at once. We were all intermittedly laughing and crying at the same time and trying to make sense of it all. Why, in the middle of the big city of Albuquerque, New Mexico, smack-dab on the ever-busy and bustling Interstate 25, did a tiny little hummingbird hover in front of my hospital window? Why there, and why MY window? For all of us who witnessed it, it was just almost too much to absorb and understand. It felt totally supernatural, like we had witnessed a small but beautiful miracle. And, to this day, I believe we did.

☉ ⊞ ☉

The day dragged on and on. I had thought that once the doctor had introduced the induction drug that labor would begin immediately, but this was not the case. The contractions came in slow, regular waves just like in an ordinary, un-aided birth. The only way I knew I was having a contraction at all was because of the monitor next to my bed. As the contractions came the machine began beeping wildly, the baby's heart rate would increase along with mine and then, slowly, the contraction would dissipate and then stop altogether. It was such a strange sensation to know that I was having a contraction and yet I couldn't feel a thing! As the contractions became more regular and close together, they moved me into another room and prepared for our baby's arrival. The time had finally come. The nurse checked to see how dilated I was and realized the baby was coming right then! I, of course, felt nothing, and was totally dependent on the nursing staff and those irritating little machines to tell me what my body was doing. SO, the baby was coming down the birth canal and FAST, so what had been an entire day of waiting turned into an emergency situation. "Don't push, Mrs. Ellis. Hold on until we can get the doctor in here!" the nurse had said. All of a sudden the birthing room was filled with people—all kinds of people. People I hadn't even seen or met yet. I asked the nurse who all these people were and she explained that it was the Post-Natal Emergency Team. "Just in case," she told me.

Well, great. That's JUST great! It was like a dog-gone convention in there! I couldn't believe it! Rich and I just tried to stay focused on each other and on the task at hand. Then the doctor made his appearance and it was almost time to push. It was time to have my baby. I almost forgot about all the strangers in the room as the doctor said, "Don't push, Robin. Don't push!" I couldn't feel anything anyway, and the doctor barely had time to put on his mask and gloves before…."There's her head! Her head is out!" Rich's mouth was wide open in amazement as he stood next to the doctor, ready to catch the baby as she came out of the womb. Then Rich said, "Honey, her eyes are open. Her eyes are wide open!" That baby of ours came down the birth canal, poked her head out and looked right into her daddy's eyes. "Now, give us one more big push, Robin," the doctor said, and out she came, right into her daddy's hands. They laid her tiny little body down on the bed between my legs, and the doctor handed Rich the surgical scissors to cut the umbilical cord. Once he had cut the cord, the Post-Natal Emergency Team of doctors swooped down and picked her up, laid her on a tiny little examining table, and went to work on her.

Those doctors took my baby away from me! I couldn't believe it! I was shocked and more than a little angry that I didn't even have a chance to see her before they snatched her up and went to work on her. Those doctors looked her over for what seemed like an eternity, and I practically held my breath the whole time. I remember the sound of Jona crying tears of joy and saying, "She's perfect, Robin. She's just perfect!" And I remember looking over at our baby, when I could muster up the strength, and seeing the tiniest little bottom I've ever seen sticking up in the air. I couldn't believe how tiny she was, and I wanted so badly to hold her in my arms and kiss her little face. But the doctors kept on working on her, looking her over time and time again, doing things that only doctors understand, and scaring me to death! I couldn't breath. I could barely look over at her anymore for fear of seeing something unthinkable, like them having to whisk her away to surgery or WORSE!

The doctor and a nurse or two were tending to my body, sewing me back together and cleaning up the wounds, and I wasn't even conscious of them. I had my eyes on my baby and the doctor's around her. After some undetermined amount of time, the doctors began to leave the room, one at a time and without a single word to me or my husband. First one left, then the next, until there wasn't one of them left in the room. At that point, one of the nurses put a little pink cap on our baby's tiny little head and brought her over to me and put her on my chest. I looked at the nurse, the nurse looked at the doctor, and then the doctor said those two words that reverberate in my soul. "She's alright!" he said. And then the nurse chimed in. "Your baby is alright, Mrs. Ellis. The doctors couldn't find one problem with her. She is perfectly alright."

She's alright! She's alright! Our sweet and tiny miracle baby is alright! I could barely believe my ears. I was crying and kissing and kissing and crying and looking our baby over from head to toe. Rich and I counted her fingers and toes over and over again. They were all there! Two eyes, two ears, one mouth, one tiny little nose. Everything! It was all there! She's really and truly alright! The room quieted down now, and it was just a nurse or two and Rich and Jona milling around, looking at our baby and cooing and crying and counting fingers and toes and then crying some more. She's alright. Praise God, she's really and truly alright....

⊡ ⊡ ⊡

It took some time for it all to soak in. I was holding our baby, our Tess Elizabeth, in my arms and, as tiny as she was, there was not one thing wrong with her. Not one thing. Now, how could that be? How could our baby be subject to an environment so toxic and inhospitable in the womb and emerge without a single physical problem? We just could not make sense of it. It was a miracle, to be sure. SHE was a miracle. I looked down at our tiny little miracle baby resting peacefully in my arms and I realized that we were dressed alike. The nurse had put a little pink cap on her tiny little head that looked very much like the pink cap I was wearing to cover up my baldness. "Like mother, like daughter," I thought, and giggled to myself. "We have matching caps on!" I said to Rich as they were wheeling us down to another room.

"Yeah, you guys are beautiful," Rich said. And we held each other's hand as they settled me into a real bed for the night. At that point the nurse came and took Tess to the nursery so that I could get some sleep. Rich went along with her and the two of them stayed up all night together, I heard. As I was drifting off to sleep, I envisioned Tess inside of my body, inside of my womb. And inside the womb there was a web of Golden Light woven around my baby. And that web of Golden Light kept my baby safe. And that Golden web protected my baby. And my baby, against all odds, was perfectly ok. All I could think of all that night were the two words the doctor had uttered. The two most beautiful words I'd ever heard. "She's Alright." Our baby is alright…. Thank you, God. She is really and truly alright.

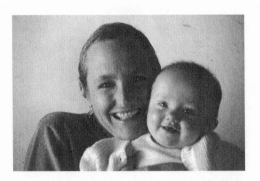

Afterword

December 2011, Alamos, Sonora, Mexico

As I sit here today and prepare for Christmas with my family in our home in Mexico, I am flooded with gratitude. Our miracle baby is now 10 years old, growing and maturing as if nothing out of the ordinary had ever occurred in her short life. I am as perplexed as I am thankful that the nightmare journey we embarked on a little more than a decade ago has had such a happy ending. Both of our daughters are healthy and beautiful and full of the love for life which you pray to see in your children's eyes. We are ever awed by the immensity of the miraculous in our everyday lives.

It took 10 years for this book to emerge out of my soul. One day in the spring of 2011, I began to record my memories of the experience of having cancer during pregnancy, and the words flowed out onto the pages with a minimum of effort. As it began to take shape, I took a trip to New Mexico, thinking it prudent to inform the "characters" in the book that they had, in fact, been written about, and that the story may be printed and shared with others. I thought it important to have their permission, so I went north seeking it. While on one of these social visits with my surgeon and friend, Dr. Stephen Cetrulo in Taos, New Mexico, he decided to perform a breast exam on me as it had been about one and a half years since my last mammogram. During the exam, he found another lump. The lump turned out to be malignant. I am currently undergoing chemotherapy for Stage 2 Breast Cancer for the second time in 10 years.

If I hadn't written this book, I may not have found the lump. I find this fact extraordinary. I must express how different the cancer experience is without having a baby in my womb, but it is just as serious. I have experienced great sadness and depression from time to time during this bout with cancer, but not for extended periods. A Bible verse keeps popping into my head and comforting me even in the deepest depths of my despair. The verse comes from the book of Matthew, chapter 14, verse 31. Paraphrased, it reads, "After the first miracle, to doubt is vulgar."

I thank God for my life—where the supernatural has become commonplace. I shall never doubt again.   *Robin Kimple Ellis*

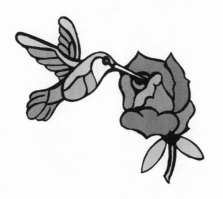

Made in the USA
Charleston, SC
11 July 2012